YOUR KNOWLEDGE HAS VALUE

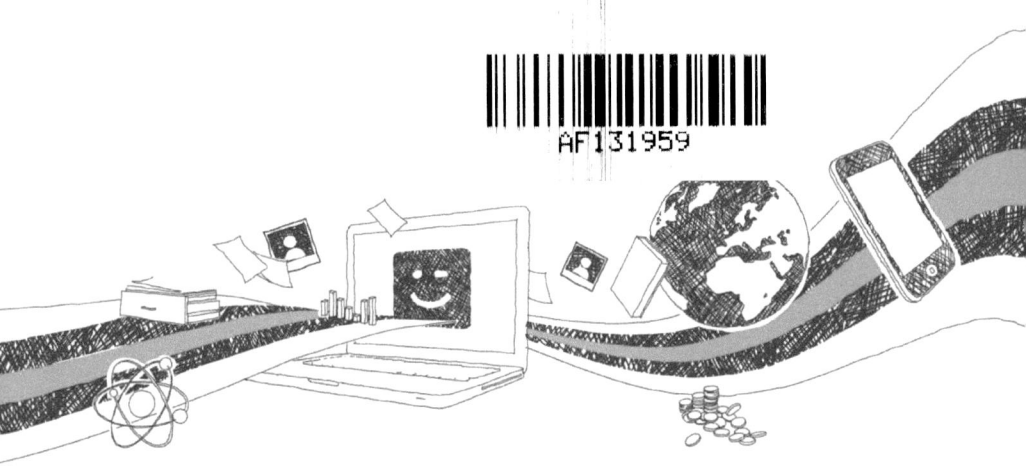
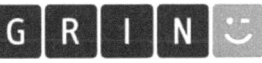

Bibliographic information published by the German National Library:

The German National Library lists this publication in the National Bibliography; detailed bibliographic data are available on the Internet at http://dnb.dnb.de .

Imprint:

Copyright © 2019 GRIN Verlag
Print and binding: Books on Demand GmbH, Norderstedt Germany
ISBN: 9783346172099

This book at GRIN:

https://www.grin.com/document/588145

Difrine Madara

Marijuana legalization. Positive and negative effects of marijuana for medical purposes

GRIN Verlag

GRIN - Your knowledge has value

Since its foundation in 1998, GRIN has specialized in publishing academic texts by students, college teachers and other academics as e-book and printed book. The website www.grin.com is an ideal platform for presenting term papers, final papers, scientific essays, dissertations and specialist books.

Visit us on the internet:

http://www.grin.com/

http://www.facebook.com/grincom

http://www.twitter.com/grin_com

Should Marijuana Be Legalised For Medicinal Purposes

Table of Contents

Introduction

Several jurisdictions around the world have passed laws legalizing the use of marijuana for medicinal purposes. These legislations allow for the use of cannabinoids and cannabis to alleviate some of the symptoms associated with terminal cancer, epilepsy and neurological illnesses (Subbaraman, 2014). However, there are serious public health concerns associated with marijuana as some experts argued that these jurisdictions have not effectively regulated its use in a manner consistent with the international drug control treaties. In many cases, Subbaraman (2014) indicated that marijuana is being diverted for use in non-medicinal purposes. In most of these countries, poor regulation of medical cannabis programmes is attributed to the low perception of risk among the policymakers and the members of the public as a whole. In the United Kingdom and several countries in Europe, marijuana is either totally banned or its use is heavily regulated. As a result, there have been increasing calls for the UK and the rest of Europe to follow the footsteps of Canada, the Netherlands, and a growing number of states in the United States where the use of marijuana for medicinal purposes has been legal for quite sometime (EMCDDA, 2020). In this regard, this essay evaluates whether the UK and the rest of Europe should legalise marijuana for medicinal purposes. This paper explored some of the positive and negative effects of marijuana on the people and the rest of the economy.

Marijuana is one of the most abused substances globally with more than 158.8 million people using it according to the United Nations. This number translates to around 3.8 percent of the global population. In the United Kingdom, around 1.3 million translating to 3.5 percent of the population had taken class A drugs in 2018 (Aguilar, Gutiérrez, Sanchez and Nougier, 2018). Among these people was 6.5 percent of 12 to 18-year-olds who were marijuana users. The above statistics showed that despite the ban on marijuana, a significant proportion of the UK population was still able to access marijuana for recreational or medicinal use (EMCDDA, 2020). To evaluate whether marijuana should be legalised for medicinal use, the author conducted a critical literature review of various studies and reports on the effects of marijuana use for medicinal purposes.

The rest of the paper is the findings of the critical literature review. These findings are organised in terms of the history of marijuana and its early uses, chemistry, and pharmacology of cannabis, the positive and negative effects of marijuana and finally a summary of the findings.

History of marijuana and its early uses

Cannabis originated in Central Asia and the Indian subcontinent. However, the first use of the cannabis plant could be traced to China and Japan, which used its fibre for fabric and rope during the Neolithic age. Though it is unclear when the psychoactive properties of cannabis were discovered, evidence of burning cannabis dates back to 3500 BC among the Romanian kurgans (Subbaraman, 2014). Historical studies also indicated that the plant was used to perform ritual ceremonies among the Proto-Indo-European tribes living around the Pontic Caspian Steppe during the Chalcolithic period (Subbaraman, 2014). These ceremonies spread to western Eurasia with the Indo-European migrations. Other studies showed that cannabis was present in the Indo-Iranian drug, soma. Iranians used cannabis due to its psychoactive properties. Nonetheless, the use of cannabis for medicinal purposes is associated with West Africa, the Caribbean, and South East Asia. Herbal medicine is thought to have been imported into Europe from these regions. Spaulding and Fernandez (2013) indicated that evidence of therapeutic use of cannabis dates back to 1000 BC in India where it was used in drink and food. The Chinese use marijuana seeds

3

as food. During the reign of Napoleon, marijuana use in pain relief and management became widespread in Europe due to its sedative and psychoactive effects.

Marijuana was used for this purpose due to its ability to induce mood and consciousness changes and help those at pain to relax and calm down. It is during this period that marijuana began to be used as a recreational drug in Europe. The 19th century is associated with the widespread criminalization of marijuana around the world. British colonies of Mauritius prohibited the use of cannabis in 1840 as they believed that it was having adverse effects on Indian indentured workers. The same ban was implemented in British Singapore in 1870. In the United States, the District of Columbia restricted the sale of cannabis in 1906 while Canada criminalised cannabis in 1923 with the enacted of the Opium and Narcotic Drug Act, 1923. In 1925, the International Opium Convention at The Hague banned the exportation of Indian hemp to countries that had banned its use and introduced a requirement that importing countries issue certificates to confirm importation indicating that the hemp is only required for medical or scientific use (Cohen, Weizman, and Weinstein, 2018).

In 1937, the production of Indian hemp was restricted through the Marihuana Tax Act. The five decades after the ban of marijuana saw increased interest in the plant from liberal lobbyists and researchers. These efforts led to the beginning of state decriminalization policies of the 1970s to 1990s to allow patients to access medical needs (Subbaraman, 2014). The cannabis criminalization trend changed in 1972 with the Dutch government classifying cannabis in a less dangerous drug category thus paving the way for the drug to be available for both medicinal and recreational uses. In 2013 and 2018 respectively, Uruguay and Canada legalised cannabis production and use for both recreational and medicinal purposes. So far, more than 20 states in the United States have also legalised cannabis use. The wave of legalization and decriminalization is based on the findings of initial studies that indicated that cannabis was less dangerous than earlier believed (Spaulding and Fernandez, 2013). Currently, 26 states have legalised marijuana use while 16 states adopted cannabidiol (CBD)-only laws, which are aimed at protecting certain strains of marijuana for medicinal uses.

Chemical structure and pharmacology of marijuana

Cannabis can be simply defined as a natural plant product that contains a psychoactive element known as tetrahydrocannabinol (Δ^9-THC). The plant is scientifically known as Cannabis Sativa L and mainly grows in temperate and tropical areas. Cannabis is one of the most widely consumed stimulants throughout the world alongside tobacco, alcohol, and caffeine (Subbaraman, 2014). The plant has also been a common source of fiber throughout history. The dried flowering tops and leaves of cannabis can also be used as an herbal drug. Recently, the use of cannabis as an analgesic has increased in clinical practice, especially in cancer chemotherapy. The most active component of the cannabis plant is the Δ^9- tetrahydrocannabinol (Δ^9-THC or simply THC), which is also referred to as dronabinol. THC exists in four stereoisomers but only (–)-Trans-isomer occurs naturally. The systematic name of THC is (−)-(6aR,10aR)-6,6,9-trimethyl-3-pentyl- 6a,7,8,10a-tetrahydro-6H-benzo[c]chromen-1-ol. The cannabis plant also contains THC related products, including Δ^9- tetrahydrocannabinol-2-oic acid and Δ^9-tetrahydrocannabinol-4-oic acid (THCA). THCA is usually converted to THC during smoking (Cohen, Weizman, and Weinstein, 2018).

Consequently, the pharmacology of cannabis is relatively complex due to the presence of multiple cannabinoids in the plant. Even at a small dosage, cannabis produces sufficient

5

cannabinoids resulting in euphoria, anxiety relief, sedation, and drowsiness. In some cases, the effect of these psychoactive substances is similar to those associated with alcohol consumption (Wilkinson, Yarnell, Ball and Radhakrishnan, 2016). When cannabis is consumed through smoking, THC can be detected in the person's plasma within seconds of inhalation. A person consumes an average of 10–15 mg of THC within five to seven minutes while the peak plasma levels of Δ^9-THC are estimated to be 100 µg/L. In addition, cannabis is highly lipophilic thus distributes easily throughout the body. After consumption, two active metabolites, i.e. 11-hydroxy-Δ^9-THC and 8β-hydroxy-Δ^9-THC and two inaction substances, i.e. 8α-hydroxy-Δ^9-THC and 8α, 11-dihydroxy-Δ^9-THC — are formed. Other minor metabolites are excreted with urine and faeces as glucuronide conjugate. The use of cannabis for medicinal purposes is supported by clinical evidence that indicated little evidence of organ or tissue damage among moderate users (Spaulding and Fernandez, 2013). Compared to tobacco, marijuana is considered to be relatively risk-free. Furthermore, fatalities associated with marijuana are rare while the causative relationship with mental health problems is yet to be established.

Effects of marijuana on a person's body

Cannabis has varied effects on a person's body in the short term and long term respectively. In the short term, consumption of cannabis leads to panic and anxiety, impaired attention, memory and sometimes it is considered to be a risk factor in psychotic symptoms (Spaulding and Fernandez, 2013). Consumption of cannabis increases the risk of accidents and the ability of the person to think clearly. Drivers with THC in their blood were found to be three to seven times more likely to cause an accident. However, studies have found no evidence of a causal relationship between THC and accidents. Short term effects of cannabis on the body can, however, be altered if it is laced with other opioid drugs, such as heroin or fentanyl. The opioids enhanced the psychoactive properties of cannabis and increased the danger of overdose. Other short term effects of marijuana consumption include the inability to concentrate and distortions of sense and time. Just like tobacco and alcohol, marijuana also has detrimental potential on a person's health by augmenting respiratory symptoms. Some opponents of marijuana consumption have also indicated that it can lead to a decrease in sperm and testosterone levels in men as well as impacting on female ovulation and premenstrual cycle (Cohen, Weizman, and Weinstein, 2018). Other side effects of marijuana consumption include fatigue, a decrease in libido and changes in body composition.

In the long term, initial studies suggest that exposure to marijuana could lead to physical, mental, behavioral and social health consequences. For instance, mothers who used marijuana during pregnancy were more likely to give birth to children who are depressed, hyperactive and inactive. Pacula and Smart (2017) suggested that chronic heavy marijuana consumption could adversely impact the respiratory system as it is associated with coughing, sputum production, wheezing and enhanced symptoms of chronic bronchitis. Nonetheless, marijuana consumption has not been associated with chronic obstructive pulmonary disease. Cannabis smoke is made up of several organic and inorganic chemical compounds that could be harmful to the body. For instance, cannabis smoke has been found to contain tar similar to the one in tobacco alongside more than 50 different carcinogens, such as reactive aldehydes, polycyclic hydrocarbons, and nitrosamines. These chemical compounds when inhaled results in an increased risk of cancer. However, the risk of lung or upper airway cancer is negligible when cannabis is smoked in small or moderate amounts. Though evidence linking cannabis with cancers is still little, in general, there is a far lower risk of pulmonary complications for regular cannabis smokers compared to

7

tobacco smokers. However, a 2015 review linked cannabis use to the development of testicular germ cell tumors (TGCTs) while another study associated lifetime cannabis use to the risk of head or neck cancer (Wilkinson, Yarnell, Ball and Radhakrishnan, 2016). Elsewhere, neuroimaging studies linked cannabis use to reduced hippocampal volume.

At an epidemiological level, cannabis use has been associated with an increase in the psychosis risk or earlier onset of psychosis. Though epidemiological association with psychosis is robust, there is still a lack of evidence of the causal relationships. Nonetheless, studies suggested that cannabis use could be a trigger to a person's predisposition to mental illness. Cannabis use is also hypothesised to be a risk factor for depression and anxiety disorder. Wilkinson, Yarnell, Ball, and Radhakrishnan (2016) also linked cannabis use to reinforcement disorders. According to studies, it is estimated that around 9 percent of people who experiment with marijuana eventually become dependent based on the DSM-IV (1994) criteria. According to a 2013 review, cannabis use on a daily basis contributed to a 10 to 20 percent rate of dependence. Cannabis dependence resulted in poor academic achievement, increased deviant behavior in children and adolescence, rebelliousness, alcohol problems and poor social relationships. Surveys indicated that among the 50 percent of daily users of marijuana experience withdrawal symptoms upon cessation. Some of the withdrawal symptoms include craving, dysphoria, sleep problems, and irritability. Based on the DSM-V criteria, 9 percent of people who are exposed to cannabis develop cannabis use disorder (Calabria, Degenhardt, Hall and Lynskey, 2010).

Positive and negative effects of marijuana for medical purposes

Positive effects

Historical studies showed that the medicinal value of marijuana was noticed back in 2900 BC in ancient China during the reign of Emperor Fu Hsi. Hsi claimed that the cannabis plant contained opposite and contrasting forces, i.e. Yin and Yang, which complemented one another to support natural systems (Pacula and Smart, 2017). Two centuries after this discovery, Shen Nung, father of traditional Chinese medicine, began to use marijuana to treat several ailments. Today, health researchers believe that marijuana has the medicinal potential to treat conditions, such as Lou Gehrig's disease, epilepsy, Parkinson's disease, multiple sclerosis, Crohn's disease, glaucoma, cancer, seizures, post-traumatic stress disorder (PTSD), chronic muscle spasms, and a wide range of terminal illnesses. In many places around the world, the health benefits of marijuana are believed to surpass its potential health risks. Due to these potential health benefits, medical use of marijuana has spread around the world with the plant components being prescribed by physicians just like any other medication (Wilkinson, Yarnell, Ball, and Radhakrishnan, 2016). However, marijuana is still approved, prescribed and availed in a very different manner compared to other commercially available prescription drugs. Though the differences in prescriptions pose numerous challenges to users and physicians, its medicinal value cannot be ignored.

One of the fundamental benefits of medical marijuana to clinicians is that it reduces the use of prescription drugs. Clinical studies confirmed that medical marijuana had fewer side effects compared to other painkillers. In these studies, the researchers observed that patients who used marijuana for medical purposes felt much better overall (Wilkinson, Yarnell, Ball and

9

Radhakrishnan, 2016). Unlike common opioids, such as morphine or oxycodone, marijuana was not habit-forming and thus was less dangerous when misused. Nonetheless, using the drugs as prescribed by the physician is the best way to ensure safety from overdose and death. Marijuana overdose and fatalities are very rare compared to other painkillers. Due to the addiction and overdose risk factors associated with opioids, national health leaders are in consensus that the use of opioid painkillers should be reduced. However, before reduction, a viable alternative must be identified. According to many studies, medical cannabis is a good replacement for opioids due to their low-risk factors and huge medicinal benefits. According to a 2016 study, researchers found that marijuana played an important role in reducing the opioid epidemic (Calabria, Degenhardt, Hall and Lynskey, 2010). The researchers found that the daily doses of painkillers dropped by 1826 doses in the American states that had legalised medicinal marijuana. Another review suggested that cannabinoids found in marijuana could help people in opioid addiction recovery. Based on this evidence, it is important to legalise medical marijuana to reduce the dependence of the nation on different forms of opioids.

Medical marijuana results in positive medicinal benefits, such as a decrease in inner-eye pressure, pain relief, nausea suppression, and vomiting and appetite stimulation. In addition, marijuana components can be used alongside other drugs to treat symptoms associated with cancer, such as pain, nausea, and vomiting, reduce multiple sclerosis symptoms, such as pain, muscle spasm, and urinary problems. Wilkinson, Yarnell, Ball, and Radhakrishnan (2016) indicated that medical marijuana positively impacts the treatment and relief from symptoms of eczema, epilepsy, Huntington's disease, and insomnia. Recent studies indicated that cannabis contained components that inhibited the growth of some cancer cells throughout the body. Though the research on the correlation between marijuana use and cancer cell growth is still at an infant stage, it is important to note that there is no study that has completely contradicted this argument. According to Professor Gregory Gerdeman of Eckerd College, marijuana has tumor-fighting properties (National Highway Traffic Safety Administration, Governors Highway Safety Association, & the Volpe National Transportation Systems Center, 2017). As a result, the use of marijuana could potentially minimise symptoms and effects of cancer or even provide immunity towards it. To determine the truth in this statement, more studies will be needed on this topic. Pacula and Smart (2017) indicated that marijuana use and the cannabis Sativa plant have the potential to assist in alleviating the symptoms of some ongoing medical conditions, including cancer and other forms of terminal illnesses. Though other studies disputed these claims, recent studies confirmed that marijuana reduced nausea and vomiting among cancer patients who were receiving chemotherapy.

Marijuana also possesses an entourage effect. The entourage effect refers to a proposed mechanism where cannabis compounds apart from tetrahydrocannabinol (THC) act synergistically so as to modulate the overall psychoactive effects of the plant. This mechanism is based on the evidence that the whole plant can provide more relief than administering some isolate compounds or cannabinoids. Though this might sound to be a trivial issue, the mechanism is a major motivator for the use of the entire cannabis plant for medicinal purposes instead of a few isolated compounds. According to proponents of the entourage effect mechanism, the cannabis plant has the potential of easing THC-induced anxiety or psychosis and their effects on a more satisfying net outcome (Calabria, Degenhardt, Hall and Lynskey, 2010). However, it is important to understand that pharmacokinetics may account for a proportion of the perceived difference in the net outcome. From this perspective, it is clear that smoking would produce more immediate effects than oral consumption of marijuana and can also ensure greater precision of dosage. On the other hand, oral administration of cannabis compounds or opioids results in a longer duration of effect thus the effect is relatively smaller compared to when the plant is smoked. In another study, cannabis smokers suffering from HIV were found to have a better caloric intake and body weight compared to nonsmokers (Wilkinson, Yarnell, Ball and Radhakrishnan, 2016). This implies that smoking cannabis leads to faster responses from the body than oral intake or any other method.

Besides, surveys confirmed that the legalisation of marijuana either for recreational or medicinal use has not led to an increase in its overall use. Critics of legal medical marijuana argued that the legalisation of cannabis could result in increased use, especially among minors (National Highway Traffic Safety Administration, Governors Highway Safety Association, & the Volpe National Transportation Systems Center, 2017). In fact, legalization has led to an opposite impact on its use due to more effective targeted regulation and awareness creation efforts. In the United States, the percentage of teenagers using cannabis has steadily dropped in Colorado since it was legalised. Furthermore, in states where marijuana is legalised, surveys indicated that the level of consumption has remained way below the national average. Legislations, such as in Florida that requires a person can only obtain medical marijuana if he or she has qualified conditions certified by a state physician for a period of time has even made it harder to obtain the drug than before. Such legislation also ensured that a person cannot obtain marijuana for the wrong reasons (Wilkinson, 2013). As a result, medical marijuana is successfully being used by mainstream practitioners in California and Florida to treat AIDS, arthritis, anorexia and cancer symptoms. In a nutshell, there is growing evidence that the benefits of marijuana legalization are immense and thus the need to amend laws to allow medical practitioners to use it for the benefit of their patients.

Negative effects

Apart from the numerous benefits of marijuana highlighted in the previous section, there are also several numerous side effects linked to the consumption of marijuana. Some of the issues outlined in relation to this include abuse issues and increased tolerance. In addition, studies have found that when a marijuana user decides to abstain from consumption, he or she may be affected by withdrawal symptoms (National Highway Traffic Safety Administration, Governors Highway Safety Association, & the Volpe National Transportation Systems Center, 2017). Other side effects often attributed to marijuana include manipulation of senses, tiredness, fatigue, cognitive impairment, anxiety, tiredness, reduced coordination, hallucinations, mood alterations, increased blood pressure and heart rate, blurred vision, and coughing, among others. Besides, studies have associated marijuana use with developmental problems among kids whose mothers smoked during pregnancy. These kids were more likely to suffer from low birth weight, anaemia, and impaired impulse, and so on. Elsewhere, studies hypothesised that marijuana consumption was positively associated with heart problems. According to Calabria, Degenhardt, Hall, and Lynskey (2010), researchers concluded that though the absolute risk of cannabis-related cardiovascular problems for healthy people is low, it can have temporary effects on the cardiovascular system of a person that uses it frequently or has other health problems.

The use of marijuana for either medicinal or recreational purposes leads to psychological and physiological dependence. According to Borges, Bagge, and Orozco (2016), consumption of marijuana will lead to neuroadaptation that can result in withdrawal effects depending on the individual and frequency of use. Just like any other addictive drug, marijuana is linked to various psychological effects during the abstinence phase. Some of these psychological symptoms include aggression, nervousness, and insomnia, loss of appetite, restlessness, and depression. A study conducted on heavy cannabis users' unmasked physical neuroadaptation, which was manifested through discomfort, stomach pain, tremors, fever chills, and headaches whenever they attempted to abstain (Wilkinson, 2013). These signs were predictive of relapse in substance abuse disorders, in this case, cannabis use disorder. Depending on the severity of the withdrawal effects, the user may experience a lack of sleep or even develop impulsive behavior. In Europe, the European Monitoring Center for Drugs and Drug Addiction (EMCDDA) estimated that at least 77 million people had used cannabis. Due to this, a significant number of Europeans were at a higher risk of cannabis use disorder (CUD) (Aguilar, Gutiérrez, Sanchez, and Nougier, 2018). Due to this, allowing the use of marijuana could make it easier for citizens to access the drugs thus leading to a potential dependence or addiction problem that would be difficult to address.

Excessive use of marijuana is linked to various mental illnesses. According to a 2016 survey conducted by the National Survey on Drug Use and Health, the researchers found that 28 percent of adults who used marijuana were experiencing major depressive episodes while 9.7 percent had experienced serious suicidal thoughts (Aguilar, Gutiérrez, Sanchez and Nougier, 2018). Overall, 24 percent of adults who attempted marijuana in 2016 suffered from a mental illness or condition that resulted in serious functional despair. Another study found that young people suffering from chronic or severe depression in early adolescence faced a higher risk of developing marijuana use disorder than young people who had fewer symptoms of depression (Wilkinson, 2013). Some of the common symptoms of depression among marijuana users included a decline in interests of everyday activities, fatigue, weight loss and changes in sleeping patterns. Marijuana is also considered to be a risk factor for schizophrenia and other psychotic disorders. Various criteria, including temporal relationship, biological gradient, biological

14

plausibility, and the epidemiological establishment of causation suggested that this relationship could be significant. However, genetic variation criteria did not fulfill this association based on strength and specificity. The study indicated that marijuana may precipitate schizophrenia in a genetically vulnerable population (European Monitoring Centre for Drugs and Drug Addiction, 2018). The study also highlighted that the use of marijuana at an earlier age increases the risk of developing other psychotic disorders.

Excessive consumption of marijuana could lead to adverse effects on cognition. Previous studies linked persistent and long periods of marijuana consumption to decline in cognition. In a data analysis of a population aged between one and 38 years, the findings supported the earlier evidence that cannabis use during adolescence led to cognitive impairment in several areas, including processing speed, executive functioning, verbal comprehension, and perceptual reasoning (Borges, Bagge and Orozco, 2016). However, these findings were criticised for focusing on populations of higher socioeconomic status and making conclusions from smaller samples. In this case, more studies in relation to cognitive decline and cannabis use were suggested. In the meantime, studies highlighted that marijuana use does not offer significant therapeutic benefits as earlier suggested. According to clinical trials to investigate marijuana efficacy in the United States, the researchers found that the effectiveness of marijuana in treating HIV/AIDS symptoms, epilepsy and chemotherapy-associated vomiting was very minimal. Similar results were found when a randomised, double-blind, placebo- and active-controlled trial was conducted to assess the efficacy of smoked marijuana and its potential implications. Wilkinson (2013) found that the effectiveness of marijuana use was superior in placebo but not in Ondansetron in treating nausea.

The recent literature review also highlighted the weakness of marijuana use in pain management and the treatment of rheumatoid arthritis, dementia, and symptoms associated with multiple sclerosis. However, these findings do not imply that marijuana components totally lack therapeutic effects. In fact, marijuana has been found to have the potential to alleviate the symptoms of various diseases (Wilkinson, 2013). What these studies suggest is that more research should be done to identify specific conditions that marijuana can be used and more evidence to justify the suggested conditions. Meanwhile, marijuana is thought to be harmful to the respiratory system of a person. Some studies have linked marijuana use to symptoms associated with obstructive and inflammatory lung disease and an increase in the risk of cancer. Studies also indicated that heavy users of marijuana were at an increased risk of reduced pulmonary function and were associated with negative effects on other organ systems, including immunologic, gastrointestinal, and reproductive systems (European Monitoring Centre for Drugs and Drug Addiction, 2018).

Marijuana use among adolescents has been increasing quite fast. According to a recent data tracking risk perception and use of marijuana, the researchers found that there was an inverse relationship between risk perception and marijuana consumption (Aguilar, Gutiérrez, Sanchez and Nougier, 2018). This finding implies that as risk perception of cannabis use continues to wane among adolescents; the use of marijuana is rapidly increasing. Among adults above 26 years old in the United States who had used marijuana, 62 percent went ahead to use cocaine at some point while 9 percent went on to use heroin. 54 percent of this group also used non-medical mind-altering prescription drugs (Aguilar, Gutiérrez, Sanchez and Nougier, 2018). This finding indicates marijuana functions as a gateway drug to other strong drugs due to low-risk perception users associated with the drug. With legalization, many critics assume that risk

16

perception will decrease the leading increase in the prevalence of marijuana consumption among adolescents. Given the negative effects of marijuana, such as cognitive impairment and onset of long term psychosis, the use of marijuana among adolescents remains a serious concern among policymakers.

Finally, marijuana use has some social safety implications for users and others. Since marijuana impairs judgment and the ability to track moving objects, marijuana users are more likely to cause motor vehicle accidents.Borges, Bagge, and Orozco (2016) confirmed that there was a positive correlation between cannabis intoxication with motor vehicle accident fatalities. Though there are both positive and negative effects of marijuana consumption on a person's health and wellbeing, more studies need to be conducted to help in making an objective decision on when, how much and what extent of marijuana should a person use. From the literature, it is evident that medical marijuana has several benefits but has dire weaknesses that call for its administration to be done under doctor's care (European Monitoring Centre for Drugs and Drug Addiction, 2018). In the cases of legalization of medicinal marijuana, it should only be done from an evidence-based perspective. At this point, the available evidence suggests that medicinal marijuana should be legalised in moderation by considering the side effects associated with heavy and frequent use.

Conclusion

The goal of this paper was to determine whether the United Kingdom should legalise marijuana for medicinal purposes. Though the plant was discovered more than 5000 years ago and was in use for different purposes, including medicinal uses in different civilizations, the use of the plant has only been criminalised in the last two centuries. The prohibition of marijuana in the 19th and 20th centuries around the world was never based on scientific evidence. However, since the 1970s, more studies have been conducted in several countries with most findings indicating that marijuana may not be as dangerous as was traditionally assumed. In fact, the plant is considered to have considerable therapeutic benefits and other medicinal advantages. For example, studies indicated that marijuana has specific compounds that could help in the treatment of symptoms of diseases, such as cancer, multiple sclerosis, and HIV/AIDS, among others. Around the world, trials and studies are being conducted to determine these therapeutic compounds and how they should be effectively administered to minimise long term health risks.

Nevertheless, clinicians have warned against the misuse of marijuana. Various studies also raised concerns regarding the use of the drug for recreational use. Though there are no robust and conclusive studies regarding the issue, many studies suggest that excessive use of marijuana could result in adverse health effects, such as addiction. A person who stops the use of marijuana could also suffer withdrawal syndrome. Besides, studies showed that marijuana consumption could have serious mental health, cognitive and respiratory problems. In this regard, legalization of marijuana for medicinal purposes in a public health and criminal justice issue. That is, marijuana should be promoted as an analgesic rather than a recreational drug. Hence, policy tools, such as registration of patients and caregivers should be used to lock out those who are seeking the drug for other purposes. However, medicinal marijuana policies should be flexible to allow for changes in the case of new findings.

References

Aguilar, S., Gutiérrez, V., Sanchez, L and Nougier, M. (2018). *Medicinal cannabis policies and practices around the world*. Available from International Drug Policy Consortium website:

http://fileserver.idpc.net/library/Medicinal%20cannabis%20briefing_ENG_FINAL.PDF

Borges, G., Bagge, C. L and Orozco, R. (2016). A literature review and meta-analyses of cannabis use and suicidality. *Journal of Affective Disorders*, Vol. *195*, pp. 63-74. doi:10.1016/j.jad.2016.02.007

Calabria, B., Degenhardt, L., Hall, W and Lynskey, M. (2010). Does cannabis use increase the risk of death? Systematic review of epidemiological evidence on adverse effects of cannabis use. *Drug and Alcohol Review*, Vol. *29*, No. 3, pp. 318-330. doi:10.1111/j.1465-3362.2009.00149.x

Cohen, K., Weizman, A and Weinstein, A. (2018). Positive and Negative Effects of Cannabis and Cannabinoids on Health. *Clinical pharmacology and therapeutics*. Available at: https://www.researchgate.net/publication/331647567_Positive_and_Negative_Effects _of_Cannabis_and_Cannabinoids_on_Health

EMCDDA. (2020). Cannabis drug profile. Available at: http://www.emcdda.europa.eu/publications/drug-profiles/cannabis

European Monitoring Centre for Drugs and Drug Addiction. (2018). *Medical Use of Cannabis and Cannabinoids: Questions and Answers for Policymaking*. Available from Publications Office of the European Union website:

http://www.emcdda.europa.eu/system/files/publications/10171/20185584_TD061818

6ENN_PDF.pdf

National Highway Traffic Safety Administration, Governors Highway Safety Association

and the Volpe National Transportation Systems Center. (2017). *Impact of the*

Legalization and Decriminalization of Marijuana On the DWI System. Available

from The National Cooperative Research and Evaluation Program website:

https://www.nhtsa.gov/sites/nhtsa.dot.gov/files/documents/expert_dwi_panel.pdf

Pacula, R. L and Smart, R. (2017). Medical Marijuana and Marijuana Legalization. *Annu Rev*

Clin Psychol, Vol. *8*, No. 13, pp. 397-419. doi:10.1146/annurev-clinpsy-032816-

045128

Spaulding, A and Fernandez, S. (2013). *Should marijuana be legalized in the United States?*

Available from the Daniels Fund Ethics Initiative website:

https://danielsethics.mgt.unm.edu/pdf/marijuanalegalization.pdf

Subbaraman, M. S. (2014). Can cannabis be considered a substitute medication for alcohol?

Alcohol and Alcoholism, Vol. *49*, No. 3, pp. 292-298. doi:10.1093/alcalc/agt182

Wilkinson, S. T. (2013). More Reasons States Should Not Legalize Marijuana: Medical and

Recreational Marijuana: Commentary and Review of the Literature. *Missouri*

Medicine, Vol. *110*, No. 6, pp. 524-528.

Wilkinson, S. T., Yarnell, S., Ball, S. A and Radhakrishnan, R. (2016). Marijuana

Legalization: Impact on Physicians and Public Health. *Annual Review of Medicine*,

Vol. *67*, No. 1.

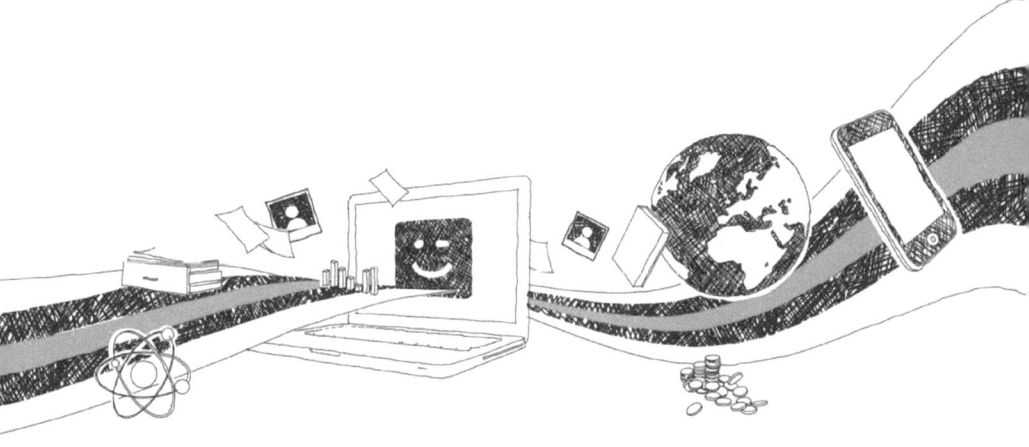
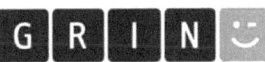